Red Pill

How to Question Reality and Conquer the Matrix

(Red Pill Mindframe and Alpha Male Strategies to Avoid Female Manipulation)

William Hardy

Published By **Elena Holly**

William Hardy

All Rights Reserved

Red Pill: How to Question Reality and Conquer the Matrix (Red Pill Mindframe and Alpha Male Strategies to Avoid Female Manipulation)

ISBN 978-0-9959965-2-6

No part of this guidebook shall be reproduced in any form without permission in writing from the publisher except in the case of brief quotations embodied in critical articles or reviews.

Legal & Disclaimer

The information contained in this book is not designed to replace or take the place of any form of medicine or professional medical advice. The information in this book has been provided for educational & entertainment purposes only.

The information contained in this book has been compiled from sources deemed reliable, and it is accurate to the best of the Author's knowledge; however, the Author cannot guarantee its accuracy and validity and cannot be held liable for any errors or omissions. Changes are periodically made to this book. You must consult your doctor or get professional medical advice before using any of the suggested remedies, techniques, or information in this book.

Upon using the information contained in this book, you agree to hold harmless the Author from and against any damages, costs, and expenses, including any legal fees potentially resulting from the application of any of the information provided by this guide. This disclaimer applies to any damages or injury caused by the use and application, whether directly or indirectly, of any advice or information presented, whether for breach of contract, tort, negligence, personal injury, criminal intent, or under any other cause of action.

You agree to accept all risks of using the information presented inside this book. You need to consult a professional medical practitioner in order to ensure you are both able and healthy enough to participate in this program.

Table Of Contents

Chapter 1: The Pill Of Truth - Red Pill 1

Chapter 2: Understanding The Red Pill .. 13

Chapter 3: The Red Pill And Its Acceptance 38

Chapter 4: Know Your Worth 48

Chapter 5: The Alpha Male - Masculine Man 91

Chapter 6: The Female Ideology Of An Alpha - A Real Man 105

Chapter 7: What Can A Lady Offer You 128

Chapter 8: Female Nature, Hyper Gamy And Female Genitals 134

Chapter 9: Attraction Level And Hyper Gamy 144

Chapter 10: The Party Girl - Setting Boundaries... 152

Chapter 11: Have No Expectations From Women 163

Chapter 12: Low Attraction And The No-Contact Rule 177

Chapter 1: The Pill Of Truth - Red Pill

Through the decades, the

The entire world is filled by men who have diminished their standards of living and the value they have. They have been coerced to act in their own wills and have denied their status as gods. They have lost their freedom to express their opinions, but are ordered to do things that are demeaning the status of men.

Who are these guys? They're all over the world. They are increasing in number and are spread across every part of the world. They are more like a woman and are classified into beta-males. They are known as SIMPS.

The red pill is available to help men get back on their feet after having become lost in the process of drinking.

If you are a man who is eager to begin the adventures of delve into female nature, and learn how their bodies are programmed in a way that is wired. This book can be an excellent resource for those who are willing to understand the truth about woman's character. Find peace with them and cease to see women as the things they're and not. Study them, repeat them and lastly, rethink the things you've learned about women since they're most likely to be a lie, and you must remain willing to accept the brutal realities of women's nature while reading the book.

Enjoy! !

Origin Of Red Pill

The source of the phrase "red pill", "blue pill" and variants thereof comes in The "Red Pill Or Blue Pill" scene in The Matrix; where the main character, Neo, is forced to choose between the red pill or take the blue pill. Red pill could allow him to discover what is really happening in the world. While the blue pill could return him to the Matrix without knowing anything.

Neo is reunited with Morpheus who offers, "Take the blue pill and everything goes back the way it was, take the red pill and experience the truth in all its ugliness." Neo is able to take the red pill and realizes that all he had learned about the world was just a truth. What he discovers isn't appealing, and can be quite difficult to swallow yet it's the truth.

What Is The Red Pill?

The red pill simply the truth. However, as you've been told, truth can be bitter. The red pill can be difficult to swallow, but I promise you, it's not the most difficult truth. It's best to learn the truth, no matter the way it is hard or how bitter it may be, than to remain fooled and lost in the deceit and lies. Even if the realization of truth is a source of anger take it in with confidence. The red pill, despite being it is bitter and hard to swallow, is a way of gaining. The red pill is a reference to gaining insight into the reality behind an event and, in particular, a fact which is hard to comprehend or that exposes negative beliefs.

To pay the price of an addict is self-destruction however the reward to the simp Red pill is liberation.

Welcome to The Red Pill. It's an arduous pill to swallow when you realize that all you've been taught and everything you've been led to believe, is false. However, once you've learned this then take it into your own mind and then begin to live the new way of life, everything becomes easier. The red pill helps you accept the real-world reality, while the blue pill can make it impossible to remain in the blissful ignorance of the illusion. TRP is a method of teaching men to become more of who they are by determining their goal to be in this world and working toward this goal, while also teaching men to find their own fulfillment.

Inhaling the red pill is the realization of reality. The pill opens your eyes and expands your perspective. Actually, taking the red pill is an acknowledgment of the futility and realisation of the absence. Contrary to that, swallowing the blue pill represents the negation of reality - depriving yourself any experience of experiencing the real truth owing to the bitterness and how hard it can be. Blue pill fantasies are a sultry one.

It's not pleasant to undergo TRP It's true that a large portion of what you find out will be a challenge to comprehend. Only proceed only if you believe in truth and not the comfort. In this article, you'll learn the skills you require to improve any part that you are in, whether you're aiming for financial success and dating a successful life, or any other thing - however, no change will be simple to achieve.

The Red pill holds a myriad of information. Do not care what people who don't know regarding taking the pill red. It's possible to label it as insensitive or sexist, however it's actually the path that will guide you through the world of a male. When you take that red pill it's not just about the comfort of your life, but you gain power: the ability to manage your own life.

The Redpill is an opposition and rejection of the bluepill . This is a skewed stance to a popular and pleasant misconception. In relation to norms of the mainstream and philosophies, it is that are in opposition to the current society standard.

The TRP program is particularly focused on "seeing reality" as it is. It is concerned with evaluating the way people act and society's functioning using a rational approach rather than an irrational belief system. The goal TRP's purpose TRP is to educate individuals about the lies and flimsy stories that have been handed through generations. TRP uncovers the elusive truth that lurks in the various facets of daily life.

TRP is not a solution to your situation, it's only an instrument. The way you utilize it will decide if you are able to transform your life to something you are proud of. It's up to you to make the right choice after learning about the red pill as well as the blue pill. TRP by itself is not moral; what you do are not determined by TRP the outcome of your actions can be considered good or not. TRP simply informs you. Let's take for instance that we know exactly the meaning of stealing and the truth is morally wrong and stealing is wrong, but when I can help protect the things I don't own; it's good. That's TRP! After having read this book how each person chooses about what to do with this knowledge is their choice. Keep in mind that sexual strategies are an act of morality. You choose what you wish to accomplish and how you'd like to do it. I think you need to be aware of the options. CHOOSE THE RIGHT PATH.

"A good workman should never blame his tools."

Red pill merely an instrument. It's not enough to know, you have to learn. When you make a mistake then you have to accept responsibility of your mistakes. If you're not finding the red pill effective for you due to the fact that there isn't a change in your attitude to living, it's the fault of you, not anyone else's. Being honest is only one of the most important aspects, but it's important to put into apply what you've learned. The learning process is not effective without practice.

There is a way to consume red pills, and be an SIMP. No whatever time you take to master TRP, why be letting the inability to achieve quick success hinder your efforts?

It's because RP takes a considerable period of time to develop, it's possible to read and try to learn TRP over the course of months but there's nothing happening and that's due to the fact that you're not relearning your old ways of doing things. Your brain is trying to replace your own beta self using the methods of the alpha. This is a slow process, but eventually you'll be there.

TRP is a process - an ongoing, steady and gradual journey it's not a goal, but this doesn't mean that you should limit yourself to a life of isolation in the process of committing to the pursuit of personal growth for the rest of your life.

The first step is to realize and accept that you're an SIMP Learn to manage your feelings and remain blunt and frank. That's the reason you're an alpha (The Red Pill philosophy is moral in the sense that it's what it is, no matter the bitter or hard it might be).

Red Pill awareness comes with an expense; reality may free you however, it does not appear pretty. -Dpsychologist

Remember that being an individual are the prize that must be snatched up, and you are the one to lead within your relationships. Be a better version of you, understand your goal and strive to achieve your goal. Develop your abilities, expand your mind and lastly, don't be a slave to.

You're the one who wins, and you're the one who owns yourself, and therefore must decide who enters your life. Beware of women who will manipulate to make you believe that you are fortunate to be blessed with them' . You should be grateful that you let them be part of your lives. The world you create, the person who is an integral part of it.

Your value is created and you decide who to give it to.

Being an Alpha You must set your goals and not the woman your primary goal. Do not play by the rules of your lady, follow your own rules. Enhance your strengths and reduce your weaknesses. You should never look vulnerable and regardless of the situation, "never be afraid to lose her".

The red pill has been around for a long time because the majority of men are unhappy. Their relationships that seem to be "just fine" are very far from being perfect. The men are giving so much to their wives and receiving much in return under the impression that simply having a part of the lives of men is all that a woman has to accomplish to be his top priority.

The men are fed up with this!

Chapter 2: Understanding The Red Pill

The ed pill's philosophy

We are here to demonstrate how to play the game, and not tell how you should lead your daily.

That's what makes the red pill a more like a philosophical concept as opposed to a religion or a religion. Religious movements and religious beliefs do not provide much liberties in relation to individual morality. They also dictate and declare with a very strict manner.

Avoid doing everything the that the red pill philosophy advises you to do. Simply, select and choose to implement what you have learn here. Be careful not to take anything we speak as gospel. Do not view it as gospel, rather as the truth (a bitter truth).

Certain men who have taken TRP attempt to adopt certain rules but are not able to accept others. This group of men is often known as "PURPLE PILL".

Consider TRP as a medication. It is prescribed for you in order to free your body from beta. The prescription requires you to consume the right amount of it and, as with other medications, it is important to not overdose. A high dose is harmful. Do it slowly. It is recommended to take an adequate amount of TRP. Don't take too much. The more you use TRP and the lower your risk of becoming sick. In the event of an overdose it can cause you to become upset and sexist. Women will be a target for your hatred, with no justification.

Knowledge of red pills does not cause harm. It is only teaching men to be aware of the real woman's nature. This is the idea that some red pillers believe is the way to stop being abused by women which may become harmful. The red pillers aren't extremists or preach hatred towards other genders. Their only goal to accomplish is to make everyone aware of the ways women manipulate you. The principle behind redpill is to increase awareness of manipulative and fraudulent practices.

If you're a red piller you need to be extremely knowledgeable to be able to discern signs and anticipate the potential outcomes of events Never be misled. Red pilling is not about screaming and blaming about how you hate women, but rather the strategies you have to beat your opponents at their own game.

The TRP program doesn't instruct that you should hate women, instead, but to appreciate them for the way they are, since they aren't changing However, most males don't understand this and that's the reason you hear them attacking and demeaning women.

Women who are abused by men when they take TRP just get unhappy with their lives and women, after discovering how they've behaved throughout the day is in fact wrong and then having seen the content of the red pill angers and turns hostile. As time passes, when they go further, they'll see there's more that yelling at women or getting angry - they're simply in the anger phase of the TRP.

It is common to take the red pill and harm your relationship in the absence of moderation. For instance, in order to keep your relationship it is essential to learn the needs of your spouse, specifically the desire for attention as well as the desire to be heard.

It is the reason that so many people take the idea of the red pill incorrectly. The first thing they do is become aggressive and hostile toward women. If you persist in showing women a rough side in spite of the belief that says "women tend to fall for who treat them bad" You're likely to make an unwise choice. It will cost you her to someone else who's going to take her more seriously.

Since the red pill tells us to that you must put yourself before ladies does not mean it is a complete disregard for women. If you pay excessive attention to them, it's not right and if you do not provide them with any attention that's also in error. A lot of everything is harmful.

In dealing with women use the Alpha-Beta scale. If you're completely Alpha, eventually you'll be unable to succeed. If you're 100 100% beta, you'll be unable to pass.

To ensure your safety, apply for safety, follow the Pareto principle. You should have 80% Alpha and 20 percent beta. There are signs that you're beta. You can't be Alpha every single day. Being an Alpha, you are able to get away with the beta-like behavior.

The Pareto Principle, named after the renowned economics expert Vilfredo Pareto, explains the following "80% of consequences come from 20% of the causes, asserting an unequal relationship between inputs and outputs". This principle acts as an all-encompassing reminder that the relation between outputs and inputs does not balance.

The common perception is that people substitute the term "red pill" for the words bitterness, hatred, brutality as well as suffering. Red pill means an emotional mastery and control, not a woman-hating attitude. Learn this, and then follow your intuition.

There's always confusion about what being red pilled is about. To be clear, a taking a red pill means giving a high-value to your self-worth as a person.

ACCEPTING AND ABSORBING THE RED PILL - STAGES OF RED PILL

THe response and acceptance

Red pill beliefs depend greatly on both the individual who is sending and receiving of the communication. Certain people see the idea of red pill to help them understand their problems and provides a framework for resolving the difficulties they're facing. Some people reject TRP completely and consider it to be an utterly flimsy nonsense or misogyny. The acceptance and willingness to accept TRP can be more difficult as it may seem. TRP is broken down into phases, which take place gradually. This is referred to as the STAGES OF red pill and is divided in five phases.

The five phases of TRP, in a variety of ways are a representation of the process that a majority of men have to go through before adopting the TRP philosophy and prepared to put in the huge commitment to align their lifestyle with what they want. You must put your traditional beliefs aside in an urn, and shift to a different way of living. It is time to let go of your old habits in order to make space for new ideas and the philosophy you're ready to embrace.

The five stages are the phases individuals go through following the discovery of that they have taken the red pill. They are encountered whenever someone loses someone close to them. However, they are extremely applicable to red pill, too.

The phases of the red pill are universal, and will be felt by all who have been experiencing the red pill's philosophies. While going through these stages it is common to spend various lengths of time focusing on each stage and each one is expressed in different ways. Contrary to what many believe The five stages don't necessarily happen in a specific sequence. There are times when we move from one stage to the next until we achieve a greater peace of acceptance.

There are many people who do not go through the grief stages according to the sequence below. That's acceptable and common. One of the most important aspects to understand these different stages is not to believe that you need to traverse each of them exactly in a specific sequence. Instead, it's much better to think of them as guides to grieving -- they help you comprehend and contextualize what you're experiencing.

The stages of life are different for each person. A few people carry their feelings on their sleeves and appear to be emotional. Some will feel their pain much more privately and display less emotions. It is important to not be able to judge the way a person feels every stage because everyone is going to experience the grief differently.

The five stages of TRP are: your denial concerning the harsh truth your anger that you experience upon discovering the truth, the bargaining that you make with the various theories of TRP The Depression you go through and finally your acceptance of TRP.

* THE DENIAL

The initial stage of awakening to red pills is the denial. It occurs after an blue pilled AFC discovers the first TRP blog or article. The first thing he notices is the feeling of denial that is an attempt to protect his beliefs. He is unable to accept that the truth is painful and difficult to accept. He isn't willing to admit that he's been operating in a false reality. First reaction when learning the facts about TRP is to ignore the truth of the situation. "This isn't happening, this can't be happening, this is not the truth, i can't believe this" many people think. It's a common reaction to explain our overwhelming emotions.

It is a typical defense method that buffers the shock of people who are confronted with the truth, especially one that is hard to digest, while also reducing the emotions. It is a way to block out all phrases and evade reality. The majority of people experience this phase is only short-term response that gets us through the initial wave of hurt.

Some blue pill-taking men who have been having gone through RP beliefs are unable to see the woman as a person who is engaged in her own program, instead they slam each other who behave in an unhonorable way.

A few of the cardinal realities of the red pill are female hypergamy and solipsism, blame shifting and the feminine penchant for manipulating and deceit are usually that which trigger the most negative reactions after introducing men on the road to red. If the red pill is indeed true then the person who took it was at fault for a lot of his troubles but it's nothing to do with be blamed on women. They simply perform their own biological and social predisposition in a predictable manner. When introduced to games before the majority of red pill theories, games can be viewed as deceitful, manipulative or moral, among others, since the gaming's enabling force alone is enough to destroy illusions. The "Denial Stage" is as well populated with the use of ad hominems to defend one's conviction system.

* "TRP is so sexist!"

* "TRP is so cynical!"

* "TRP is so delusional!"

* "Women aren't like that! They're people just like everyone else!"

* "That's mysoginy"

* "I do not believe in anything about the claims. Take them as an entire group You'll be sure to get the best one!"

If someone is going through the denial stage no matter what evidence to them of the contrary the beliefs they hold and they won't change. If you are aware of people who do this, then it's better to get over it and stop trying to persuade them.

Denial is resulted from a variety of unconscious views which stem from the belief that people have no value in nature and their total contribution to humanity is the result of their success. They must make grand shows of value, increase their worth and gain the money women get to exist. The fact that no woman can ever be as loyal to him as he hopes of love but that they are actually unable to experience this kind of love. It is a fact that the life he leads is a constant struggle and performance, if he is determined to achieve his goals as well as the fact that what said to him that he can get only came as the result of his hard working.

* ANGER

The term is usually called"the "Red Pill Rage" stage. The stage is marked by a strong feelings of anger at the society, towards women and even at the world as a overall. When the effects of masking denial start to fade the reality of life and its hurt come back, resulting in the emotion of anger. This intense emotion gets pushed away from the vulnerable part of us, then redirected, and expressed as anger. It is directed at women as well as the world in general - at womanhood all over the world for the depraved sexual plan that is known as "Alpha Fucks/Beta Bucks", at dads who aren't "raising them right", as well as at the entire world for not educating them.

Denial can make us feel guilty, which leads us to become even more irritable. It is an instinctual reaction. As a result, an individual may end up having feelings of being misled and, in addition to the people without faces, as well by the people in whom he is most confidence.

"Anger Stage," also known as the "Anger Stage" is rife with various comments, including:

* "Women are such sluts!"

* "Society is so full of sh*t!"

* "The media just LIES to everyone!"

* "WTF! B*tches are all like this! They have no honour, no loyalty, and they don't really love anyone but themselves! Fucking c*nts!"

"Anger Stage. "Anger Stage" is one which is usually short and full of intensity. If one fails to overcome the victimization aspect the stage could go throughout the years which can lead to aggressive offenders. The people who cannot keep their emotions in check in this phase become sexist and have little concern or regard for women.

It is important to remember that grieving is a private procedure that is not a time limitation, and there is no "right" way to do grieving.

* BARGAINING

When a person begins to admit to that the "red pill truths," the person will seek to compromise against the premise that is laid out, and often take a few of the elements, while denying other aspects.

The normal response to feelings of vulnerability and helplessness can be a desire to gain control by reciting an array of "If only" statements, like:

*If only I'd discovered the truth earlier.

* If only the world would not have lied to me.

If only I had not duped.

It is a way to bargain, and also a method to safeguard our minds from the realities we face. The feeling of guilt is often associated with bargaining. It is easy to conclude that there is something to have changed which would help us in the situation we're facing.

The negotiation stage may be one of the most intriguing, as it is where you find the purple pill. completely aware about the nuanced nature of the red pill thinking, the person is unable to let go of the fiction provided by the blue pill. It is interesting that this an old-fashioned idealization and characteristic of blue pill thought appears to go unnoticed, due to diverse biases. Negotiating is difficult, because dreams of taking a blue pill is deep-seated in men's minds, and the dream that they are fed in their childhood.

"Bargaining Stage," also known as the "Bargaining Stage" is typically depicted by remarks such as:

* "Not all women are like that!"

* "Hypergamy only affects some women!"

* "Yeah, people care about looks, but personality matters too!"

* "If I work real hard and learn all the pickup moves, then at least I'll get laid."

The bargaining phase is the final stage at which individuals still hold on to their blue pill belief system. Determined not to fall into the trap of letting their old beliefs collapse, they hang the last vestiges of it they consider acceptable.

* DEPRESSION

The phase of this usually lasts longest. There is a deep sense of despair and denial about life when one realizes that he's been duped, deceived and deceived by society as well as others.

At times, it's the situation that people often find themselves trapped in. They aren't convinced that they can change their lives, and they don't think it's worthwhile to attempt it.

This is characterized by remarks such as

* "What's the use? All the Chads will just get the girls anyways."

* "Make more money? Yeah, so the Chads can smash my wife on the side."

* "All girls cheat. What's the point of even getting a girlfriend?"

* "Getting laid by shallow, obnoxious women has become dull and unrewarding. And there's no sense looking for a unicorn. Maybe i'll just be MGTOW for a while."

Depression comes in waves and is derived because "unplugging" requires that all previous fantasies be put aside in the same way as.

This phase is characterized by an lack of understanding which is extremely depleting. After letting go of their feelings they will be able to proceed to the next stage, acceptance. The process can be facilitated through simple explanations and affirmations.

It's common for men to slip back into bargaining phases, as well as occasional visits to outrage. In this stage, the awakened state is akin to staring at the bottom of an ocean while one takes on the demon, and then reevaluates all aspects of the concept of.

* ACCEPTANCE

It's the state which we all strive to come to. It's characterized by calm peace, and a recognition that the universe is exactly as it is. No thought or feeling can alter this.

The ability to reach this level of TRP is which isn't accessible to everyone. Being aware of the harsh truth can occur suddenly and unintentionally, and it is possible that we will never be able to see beyond anger or denial. The phase of grief is characterized by calm and apathy. This is not a phase of joy and should be separated from depression.The ideal thing to do in this phase is to to be able to feel the pain when it is affecting your body. Doing anything to avoid it can delay healing's natural process.

Acceptance of this pill an ongoing choice that needs to be confirmed It is also extremely easy to fall back into routines. The acceptance of the red pill implies the person accepts the man will forever be expected to take care of and companion of women to the detriment of others. Refusal of this unstated basis of society will usually cause social criticism. Anyone who chooses to pursue his personal improvement, not the well-being of women or his friends, can face huge amount of disdain and ridicule.

It is important to remember that the majority of people are involved into blue pill conditioning particularly those who have the highest stake in it as well as women who are the biggest users of the program.

"Acceptance" stage is the "Acceptance" stage is marked with the following remarks:

* "I'm going to improve my life and try to find a loyal woman."

* "Even though not all girls are loyal you can still screen hard and find a decent one."

* "Yes, cheating is a possibility, but if you guard your family and your life, you can drastically reduce its odds of happening."

* "Women aren't bad. My expectations of them, and theirs of me were based on faulty premises. They are creatures of instinct, just like I am but of different instincts. If I learn what those instincts are, and teach them about mine, we can develop realistic expectations of each other and get along just fine."

The acceptance stage is considered to be the most important stage, as it is the only way to be a part of the red pill philosophy without the often tense emotions that are associated with the idea (anger depression, sadness, etc.).

Chapter 3: The Red Pill And Its Acceptance

* General View Of TRP

Do not discuss the

Red pill is available freely. The world we live in is an era of blue pills.

Something you've seen is how public views the notion of the red pill. And the way it views males who claim to be alphas with a sense of contempt. Our society is brimming with women who have changed all things to their advantage. Women are favored by society. The ideas of the red pill are met with admonishment and ridicule because they are a challenge to the norms. TRP's ideology TRP is in opposition to the feminist culture that we live in as a society.

The red pill is regularly attacked for "hating" women. TRP doesn't hate women, TRP just sees women for who they are and their behavior and behave, and according to their behavior. The bottom line is that TRP is not a feminist. and women. TRP simply doesn't respect women. They give an excuse after reason to for not doing so.

Society doesn't take note of male weaknesses. Society will only be concerned about women when they are beautiful or strong woman. Women are more likely to receive assistance whenever she's in a position of need of assistance, compared with their male counterparts. The society will always provide an insurance plan for women. White knights will come in and the government will offer and provide. For men, there is the same privileges, but your potential and capacity to increase your more power is higher than women's, but your capacity to fall off the cliff is more prominent too.

Our society has turned into an increasingly feminist one. The president can't be elected without submitting to feminist discourse and paying tribute to them. The public doesn't care any thought to the fact that you are male. The system favors women. If you consider the way society treats cases of paternity issues and divorces in favor of women (neglecting whether the allegations are fraudulent or if women are in the wrong) you'll realize how screwed by the system.

Most laws have been designed in a manner favoring women. When it comes to rape and domestic violence, the accused are believed to be guilty until proved innocence. In the event that are false allegations, women are not punished and when the accused are unable to prove innocence, their whole existence is destroyed.

The courts tend to favor women when it comes to divorces. The majority of men pay the child support and alimony throughout their lives due to the fact that they put in hard work for your career, and then achieved it while the wife decided to remain a home mother.

Men lose custody of their children in 86.8 percent of cases, and have to pay Alimony in 97 percent of instances. The system of justice doesn't guarantee that the child support funds are used by the child and not the mother.

Women are the majority of divorces. Half of weddings end in divorce and cheating women are 50% of the time, which means the chances are that it's not the fault of you, but you could have to forfeit half of your savings and pay an ex-wife a sum of money throughout your existence. If you're raped by a woman who was older than you when you were a teenager when she became pregnant, you'll have to make child support payments after you turn age 18. The rape of a man is not thought of as a crime, although men have been raped every day.

Male victim of domestic violence is nearly absent compared to the female victims. If a woman is treated by an unpopular man, he is questioned what happened in order to cause her behavior to be so ugly, however if an individual treat another in a negative way, they have decided that he's an inhuman being without any further research. If a woman is slapped by on a man, then the man is an unclean person. However, when a man hits women, they are an unfit person for hitting her. This creates a dual standard within the culture. Men's violence is often employed for humorous purposes in the media, but if the depiction of violence against women is to make a point it will trigger an intense reaction.

It is a requirement of society to have equality between genders. However, it's only not limited to the best parts like equal pay, the right to nakedness and equal representation in high pay positions. They aren't able to do so as the weight of responsibility becomes a factor - sharing costs, equally remuneration of dangerous occupations like mining, standing in the buses and trains when seats aren't readily available. In essence, women are looked upon as delicate snowflakes. And the notion of masculinity remains. Women receive an advantage regardless of whether they've done wrong and have justifications used to justify any wrongdoing. However, no natural courtesy is given to males.

It is a privilege that women enjoy by which they are able to enjoy even in the courts their punishments are less severe in the event that they're penalized at all.

* Female View of TRP

Like I said earlier Do not discuss the red pill publicly as the public is pilled. Take the red pill, but don't show women that the pill you're taking. Distinguishing the source of your power is a way to show the power. Women are not a fan of the idea of the red pill, but they adore men who demonstrate the same ethos - Alpha males. Women do not like the fact that males no longer conform in accordance with their demands. They aren't happy that we are aware of the truth.

Do not mention the pill in a way that women would be interested Just take it as a habit. The women hate the idea however they love the results.

The women are clearly against it since it exposes the weaknesses of their beliefs and behaviour such as solipsism, preferred status in law, preferential work policies, as well as an assured floor set by the federal government that is funded through wage garnished, alimony as well as child support funds which are taken out of the pockets males. They are at a disadvantage to admit it, and so they battle the issue with their wits and attempt to make it appear as a term or symbols that females and males view as negative. They refer to it as "creepy, nasty, hateful of weak males and others.

Women conceal their goals to subjugate men in the in the name of the concept of feminism. Women claim to want equality, however what they really are seeking is power with no accountability. They would like male and female privilege to be combined in one place, thereby resetting the balance of gender. They would like the advantages as women (privilege that includes being economically supported, having advantages based on appearance and being protected from physical harm from others) in addition to male privilege (authority and the respect of having a job as well as the freedom to not be assessed so severely due to appearance, etc.) that is not practical and realistic. Furthermore, it overlooks the biological foundations of how gendered perceptions of each and assumes of "everything is a social construct!" And we're all "the same" when quite it is not true.

Red pillers are a scourge to women. They view us as a threat to their beliefs. Redpillers pose a risk to women due to the fact that he's learned how to get past their supergamy and games of manipulation. Therefore, he will be using women instead of using them.

Feminism as institutionalised as it is in society is responsible for exacerbating female narcissism, encouraging them to monopolize and exemplify their worst traits (hypergamy/entitlement and solipsism) to scapegoat us collectively (as men) for their own material betterment.

Chapter 4: Know Your Worth

* You Are The Prize

You could be the one to win her prize.

Lucky to have. We are blessed to have men like this. Being a man is an accomplishment that you can feel proud of. Your achievements are the most important and all women should feel blessed to be a part of your life. It's not a ploy to be misogynistic It's the truth. Men, you deserve to be revered by a woman just because that you're a man.

In the entire world in the world, betas make up the vast majority. The term "betas" in this case will be men who do not use the red pill since the majority of red pillers are not Alpha. They are known as simps due to the fact that they are convinced that women possess higher value than men do. The world would become a more peaceful place when men realize their worth. They should not get angry for women with no worth mentioning. Don't allow yourself to be affected emotionally by a woman to perform a petty act in order to please her. As I have said before to keep the attention solely on yourself. Women don't have the ultimate goal but your goal is what matters. Woman is only an attachment, or friend on the adventure. She is either with you or in. Don't stray from your goal to earn the love of a lady. Keep your eyes open.

The most important thing about taking the pill red is that it allows you to develop into a high value male - an Alpha male. A man of high worth is one who feels comfortable in his own space He doesn't seek the attention of women. A man of high worth is one who constantly strives to become a better person and an even better person. The most important thing is knowing that the happiness lies within you, and is not tied to any woman in any way.

Women move on and off But YOU will be forever. Your attention must be focused at you since you're the winner.

One way to get an individual woman agree to be with you when it comes to relationships or anything else is to walk away. Make her feel valued in knowing that you are able to leave anytime. When you let her know that you are able to leave, she'll be willing to accept. For a male the most powerful thing you have when it comes to women isn't your money and definitely not your appearance. It's the power of your personality and your ability for keeping her on feet and show her that even if you're not telling, that it's always possible to leave! Don't take it in with her rudeness as well as her complaints and negative attitude. Although it may sound counter-intuitive you can use it to your advantage in dealing with females.

A thing I find very irritating is when a man decides to become a man of high quality and take a lower price. Women will not accept anything less. Do not attempt to overcome barriers and hurdles to please her. Do not sacrifice your hopes and happiness, your hope or your destiny just for the sake of a few crumbs of sexy.

The reason for this is that women do not comprehend the meaning of honour and sacrifice. Women are influenced by emotions in the present but if the current time is not stable, the sentiments that make them happy could be at stake. These can be very difficult times from the perspective of a male.

The prize for men is to be taken home. Being the male leader they are your most important prize - one that each woman must strive to get. Be aware of you, work on your character and women will appear to your. An overbearing man seeks power. This can cause arousal, respect and even fear among women in addition to his masculine power. Women who are weak chase men and this can lead to the eroding of trust, and parasitic relationship as an consequence of his feminine energies.

The more readily you're accessible (physically emotionally financial, physically, etc.) to women more she will not admires and respects you. the less worth you have and she'll stop taking seriously.

It is necessary to drink water and you don't require gold to survive - yet it is more expensive because of its rarity. The value of gold comes not only from utility but also the scarcity.

Don't become a simp that does not know what he is worth, thus, is prone to giving excessive focus to females. Simps don't have a life of their own, and they seek approval by women. They're too sweet and will do anything in order to please women so are happy which is why they're deemed to be dumb.

It is not appropriate to be a slave that mingles with a crowd of women. Make sure you do not engage in any of his practices and follow these rules. Because they're only to enrich his fortune and are likely to flee after he's no longer money to be sucked up. Beware of him, because the burdens he'll endure are a lot for his shoulders, he'll be on his own. The wise will be rewarded with glory but shame is on fools.

* Don't Lose Your Respect To Women

Women will never admire a man that she is able to take over and manage. Nature despises weakness. In the event that a person displays his surrender to the unconscious judgment of nature and declares to the nature's programming its inability to defend her, and also the risk that she might not reproduce properly and stay in the pattern.

It is impossible to force an individual woman to be respectful of your. The way you frame your thoughts and present your ideas is how you gain respect. A woman's shouts in order to make her respect you can make you appear to be physically abusive. Avoid doing so.

The power of boldness captures the eye and thoughts of women. You must be unapologetic when you interact with females. Be bold and take social risks. brave decisions. Women aren't enthused by those who behave like a dick, and does not have confidence to chase what he's looking for.

• If someone could guide you on the right path and then not follow through, she'll lose respect towards your.

* If you try to chase her, she'll get rid of respect for her

If you are apathetic all her dramas and petty arguments, she'll be less tolerant of you.

If you set your daughter on the pedestal she'll lose respect to the person you are.

If other women don't like you, she'll be less likable to the woman who is not interested in you.

* If a woman appears to be more emotionally strong than you are, she will have less respect for you.

If you display weaknesses, she'll be disregarded by her.

* If you fail to manage the relationship, she is likely to lose your respect.

* If you aren't a person with the drive or ambition her respect will diminish towards her.

* If you start to become dependent and dependent, she'll be less tolerant of you.

* If you are able to say "yes" to everything she claims, she'll lose respect for you.

* If you fail to adhere to the rules her respect will be diminished towards her.

If she does not believe that she can have a better future together with you, she'll begin to drop respect for your.

* If you don't manage to leave, she'll be less respectful of you.

* Never Fear Women

Don't be afraid (SCARED) about women, but be cautious of women.

It may seem contradictory however don't let me get it wrong. If i talk about fearing women do not mean having a fear of women. For this reason, the fear of being cautious (staying on guard and displaying a sense of caution concerning potential risks or challenges) so that you can avoid being manipulated by females. This is a tactic that is used to ward off women's predatory tendencies.

Men, do not fear women. Being afraid of women can be like making them look good and reducing the masculinity of men. It's unsettling to observe how many men, after taking the red pill are scared of women. They make a situation which presents women as godlike and need to be fearful. The fear-based tactic must be absconding with. Fear can be a powerful emotion which can become an impetus for self-destruction. The fear of women could cause you to be hurt. This is contrary to what you've been taught about the tenets of TRP.

The fear-based tactic comes as an outcome of the experiences that men go through of being sexy by women, a process known as the emasculation. It is the act of depriving men of their masculinity, or his male identity. That is, to make him feel inadequate or unworthy of being "manly" enough.

Use your wisdom and be cautious of females. As it was reported during the past that lips of an odd woman will drop honey and her mouth is more smooth than oil. But ultimately, she's sharp as wormwood and bitter like a double-edged sword.

THE GAME OF FEMALE MANIPULATION

The average person

Inexperienced and ignorant and. The woman's mental model is far more extensive than that of what an average woman hopes to. The reason is not because of him because his biological makeup deceives his body, and the society lied to his face, and the deck is full. However, reality is.

The perfect female manipulator can be a fascination to look at. She is able to hold men at her call. She can do this since she's taken time to study the psychology of men and how they behave so that she can effectively predict the way they react in various scenarios. She's meticulous about her actions and performs this move without even a trace suspicion. Many men do not even realize the difference when they're manipulated. The mind is the only thing that can be controlled.

Women are manipulators. They are always looking to control the person they are manipulating. The mind of theirs is always working using their femininity to convince you to make choices that favor them.

Over the years, women have mastered manipulative techniques in order to get men to obey what they want to do. Drama is a favorite for women, which allows them to use emotions to push their agenda. They are deprived of emotions, and they're not able to fight. An emotional woman is likely to be desperate to continue her mental assault. This is why she'll try to bring it back from the grave, focusing on exaggerated experiences as well as manufacturing concerns so that she can maintain the rage necessary for sustaining the psychological violence.

They are experts in this particular act, and have refined an ability that can be utilized for sexual purposes. Women have a right. It's a given that all women are entitled, and even though some women aren't the majority are. This isn't a matter of "is she entitled?" instead, it's a matter about "is she not?" Rarely will a woman express respect for the efforts of a man. Do you have a concern that she wants you to solve? The request isn't really a demand, it's a request. For her this is your duty instead of your decision to assist her. It is not a way to earn the respect, recognition or gratitude when you help entitled women since their narcissistic tendencies make themselves as deserving of. The woman may be taught from this behavior and if she's not she'll default to this behavior.

Women aren't very aware of this and usually aren't aware of and often.

Do you pay for the bill? This is what you're expected to pay the bills!

The last funds in your account to satisfy the needs of your client? You're expected to perform!

You buy her the latest and expensive mobile on the market? You're expected to make!

What if you could forgive her past filthy and shady life? Being a male is supposed to be mature and understanding and that's the right thing to do!

A bitter pill? The truth is out there and it's the most crucial aspect.

Women play men like Mozart played piano. Men manipulate nature, women manipulate men. Men have been controlled emotionally by women and to make them feel happy and accept their deceit as true. Anyone who has been influenced by his emotions regarding women's affairs will be destined to fail!

Blessed is the one who is able to read what women say as they dissect their language and find their hidden meanings.

The men have been tricked to become the primary provider. Men, as a rule, have to take care of the woman, even if she is earning well (or more so, even when they earn more than you but you still have to be able to help). So sickening!

Women are able to use men as many times as they accept to be used, but giving him nothing back. Focusing on the desire for affection that a man has and she is unable to return. Instead of being honest and truthful and letting person she's interested in know that she's not attracted, she uses the attraction to gain personal advantage. Some women try to claim they're genuine romantically connected and that everything is always one-sided (a uncommon arrangement) however, in truth she is able to label him an uninteresting sexy guy - an ORBITER. One who is constantly in and readily available for her and is just a phone or a call away, willing to do every favor she requires. What's friendship? That's an act of exploitation! In particular, if she thinks to be treated as if "she's the woman" but she doesn't reciprocate. Anyone who considers women his top first priority without taking into consideration about his health or financial current situation is undoubtedly a SIMP. Woe betides him.

Females have a method of telling men that they are doing things that are against their own will. A man may think he's doing her a favor and she'll appreciate her more. But you have achieved her status by upgrading it and elevated her to a higher status than your expectations. Don't make the same mistake again Don't make that mistake again!

It is her ability to gain from you, and not be obligated to meet the needs of you causes her be disregarded, and the loss of attraction is usually communicated through feminine language, such as " the spark's just not there anymore" and, consequently, she's likely to start to repeat the cycle with another male.

Every woman is naturally manipulative; they are able to deceive, manipulate, or lie and manipulate men throughout their lives. This includes family as well as friends. The simp may see this as normal, but an Alpha considers it to be exploitation and always ask the motive behind this self-centered curiosity.

There is a simple answer, women lack a sense of morality (sense of morality, right as well as wrong). It is only their perception or belief that it's wrong when others women oppose they are against it. In addition there is no any sense of what is right or right or wrong. So long as they feel appropriate and is good. It's what they do.

The main reason women could force a man to raise the child of another man (her argument is that it's not a sin). A man can be manipulated by a woman to let her be who she is, and let go of her history. By manipulating the idea that "a real man should do blah blah blah"

An extortionist will try to convince you to invest your money and time in a way that will not feel guilty, selfish or devious because doing this feels extremely good and just to her. It doesn't matter which way you view it as it is her turn to be on the other end of the spectrum.

Women aren't happy that men have been enlightened and red pilled. They are aware that men who have been red pilled aren't going to be able to resist their manipulative tricks. They are the reason why they hate those who take red pills. Everyone hates competition. require men to be ignorant and ignorant about their character (being the red pill) as getting red pilled implies placing yourself in the front, putting your self before other women. If women can see that you be a safe haven, they're in pain. Women can't take advantage of you since she's aware of your ability to anticipate her actions and strategies.

If you are able to recognize and expose the tricks used to manipulate you the woman feels frightened and reacts with indignation. Once she's no longer able to influence you, she calls you as the liar or the one who hates you, racist, hypocritical, sexist, and many other names that make you look shameful. You should be proud when someone calls your name in any way because it proves that you're an ALPHA.

The fact is that so long as you're a male, the women who are around you ready to leverage them to reach their objectives.

There is no woman who's exempt including your mother. This is the reason your mother will make you cherish her more than father. To ensure that when you need your way in the future, you'll take the care of her first. and she will need your help to be her advocate in the near future. manipulative.

The manipulative women are referred to as prey-type women. The term "predatory" refers to a woman who exploits men or pounces on them to gain personal advantage. The majority of women initiate of divorces once they've taken the status, money or other resources from their male victims and another (a more prestigious male) is attracted to their attention.

Have you seen how a girl can turn a man from an millionaire to a zeronaire? A man is emotionally irritated enough that he begins to lose his sense of sanity? This is a predatory impulse working.

She'll never forget what the man did to aid her climb, and will attribute the credit for her achievements her own self-esteem while transferring the blame for her shortcomings to her father.

They don't feel any guilt. For them, it's simply being female. They do not feel guilty and never be considered guilty. The desire of a woman to stay unrepentant for all time and plays an important part in her determination to create a picture of innocence. In defense, the principal method of manipulation is her pretense of innocence but offensively it's the attractiveness of her body.

The mistakes of women are never a factor but a man's errors are erased.

It is a practice that is in place within the society that allows for the exoneration and justification of her actions. Responsibility and accountability are not a thing from the world of women.

Sexual weaponisation as well as the flimsy portrayal of crying, the fake appearance of innocence and the inability to blame are methods used by women to deceive be aware of what they really are.

* The Common Strategies Of Female Manipulation

-Sudden Show Of Affection And Praises.

Then it's like she's always praising you while making you feel appreciated. She makes you feel pampered and like you're her most prized possession she has ever had in her life. The mind starts to go through the motions and you begin to think you're the best guy ever. This isn't like saying that a person deserves praise does not harm anyone. It's not even a problem. It is an important methods of expressing appreciation, and people like to be admired.

If you look closely, however, you will observe that something is different about the frequency of praise has increased. In these instances it is important for an alpha male to be able to discern the sudden show of affection and be on guard since that's the time she'll make an offer that you may have a hard time turning down, without feeling guilty. The woman is working hard and relying on this emotion perspective. She's aware that it's effective and should you too. Also, she encapsulates it all with a call to your pet's name. She'll make you think she's mad at the way she treats you. To her this is a lot greater than the fact that. She is able to turn his pet's name to an effective and profitable application. She is able to sing his name an extremely soft and gentle way. She knows exactly how to whisper it to his ears. At the same time she is watching and attentive like a dog that is ready to listen to his master's voice.

-Crying

It's not a pleasant sight to witness an emotional or crying woman particularly a beautiful woman who you have a connection with. This is incredibly heartbreaking because they appear fragile and vulnerable. She is manipulative and is more than willing to utilize the situation to advantage when you allow her to. She is aware of how emotional it can be. You think that men don't have emotions? I'll tell you why; they are emotionally charged, however they've been taught by society to conceal their emotions.

There's only one option to keep a lovely woman from crying, and especially those who mean an important thing to you. You surrender. It's not obvious yet, but she's looking at you with a smile. In fact mothers know how to make the most of this technique to their advantage! Bitter truth right?

-Comparing and Coercing

If she's looking to do things according to her own way, she could employ this approach. It isn't a direct way to make requirements, instead she'll inform you that you did the exact same thing with other individuals. Don't you get it? The woman is telling you she's not happy to be marginalized! Then she'll explain that men also are doing it to women.

You know what? It's effective! is because a lot of males, in particular aren't keen on being judged as different from others. The pressure can be overwhelming in their own bowels when your flaws will be exposed to you. The chances are it's going to be a disaster in the event that other women appear in the open and the sole woman who is not the most popular woman, and that is due to your. It isn't the best idea to make a man thought of as the stingy one that isn't able to offer "such a simple thing" for his wife. It is an excellent chance for a man to be enticed and to avoid the whole thing, he could simply have to concede.

-Obedience And Submissiveness

If you're a woman looking to be able to control her partner knows it is among the most efficient methods to convince him to listen to her demands. What a man really wants is an obeying and submissive woman who respects him and lavish him with affection. He would rather not have to be a household boss. If a woman acts in obedience to her partner this increases the likelihood of obtaining what she needs from him via persuasion 10 times. They become submissive at once and performs actions she usually would not do to try and manipulate him to do her favor in the future.

-Avoiding

You may begin to look at her, and she will try to avoid her. It will be apparent that there seems to be a gap in between you, and you'll begin to think about what that you're doing wrong or right. She understands what you're feeling and exactly what she's trying to get you to be feeling. She is playing mental games with the person you are. Most people consider something valuable when they're close to losing the item. Thus, when she presents herself in such a way, she's giving you a warning that you're about losing her. If she is able to become the "one in a million" and you're getting into serious problem. It is possible for this silence to result in a major emotional breakdown. Thus, the use of this type of trick is usually the riskiest.

-Nagging And Bombarding

Men often complain about women constantly nag their wives. This is a huge stress on the male and often the only method to force her to stop is accepting her words of rage. Another type of nagging may result in constant bombardment of the person's life, in any way she is able to. It could come in the form of frequent texts, phone calls or emails. It is possible that she will continue doing this until the person has the option of recognizing that she is an annoying person and to give in to her requests. If you're not aware that nagging can be an effective tool to get your desired outcome since the person is exhausted of hearing the same complains, the same demands or the same tale.

-Seduction And Touching

The impact of the touch of a woman is not to be underestimated. She can influence her to accomplish things that she wants without being conscious by simply touching your. Women are naturally gifted because they are able to be touched by a male, even when they are in public. Only the person touching them will realize the touch was distinct. An expert female manipulator understands the best way to approach her man and the length of time she'll permit the touch to endure while expressing her intentions through her eyes. By manipulating this way, the man will be and a victim of her whims!

The most effective weapon they have they have is, of course, their gorgeous body. By revealing a little meat here and there or kissing him in a swarm, women can make men with blood red flowing through their veins lose control. This is especially true when the person isn't self-controllable. She could give you the enticing "under the eyelashes" look and then you will receive attractive and lust-inducing messages in one go without being dependent on anyone else to figure things out.

Females are capable of succeeding with this since they understand that the natural world has cursed men with a single ailment: an insatiable need for sexual pleasure! In most cases, seduction is an early precursor to sexual sexual intimacy. As long as a male believes that he will to be able to satisfy his cravings in the course in the end, he may be uninterested in what the woman has to say regardless of whether it might be a bit absurd for him at an earlier time.

-Sex

This is the best approach. It is the most secure of all. women who are able to navigate around this tactic will keep any man under control. It's because, regardless of whether the guy does not feel he likes your style, he'll not feel the need to rescind this invitation. This means that the woman will be able to get another chance to manipulate her partner and make her case often until the moment it's done! The women who use sex to manipulate their partners, because it's their ultimate weapon, and, often, their sole option.

Sexually based manipulation is a common strategies to influence males. Women believe that, so long as there's testosterone in the world, males will want to have sexual freedom and females know how utilize it to influence men since they're the keeper of sexual the sex.

It's easy to bring your body into submission and control in removing the cause of your sexual cravings. Every sexual desire begins with our thoughts. It isn't like we get hot at once. It's an internal process. You are thinking about how wonderful it feels when you touch someone which triggers your desire for sexual intimacy that in turn boosts the testosterone level, giving you an overwhelming desire for sexual intimacy.

Let me prove this idea in a real manner. If your sister is naked while you're around and you aren't feeling anything in any way. Even worse, you are irritated at the nakedness. It's not like you feel sexual desire since you do not "think about her in a sexual way" being aware of the truth that incest is the most unclean thing to do. The fact that you don't think about her in this kind is not going to have any influence on your brain (sexual desire). Your body is unaffected by any testosterone raging since the cause (thinking this way) does not exist nor will it ever be in the form of your sibling.

The idea is simple. If you want to be a controlled male, you must control your thought process. The look of a woman in a skimpy dress is likely to make you feel hot when you think of her sexually. If you think of her the same manner as you do your mother, then her skimpy skirt doesn't matter to you as it does not affect you. The source (your thoughts) which triggers your desire isn't there.

If you're not in control of your mind, ladies will manipulate you with ease using the sex . They will know that you'll be a victim on the spot because you've got zero self control. The man with the red pill that has controlled himself and his emotions cannot be influenced by any scheme to manipulate women. He is a thinker who doesn't work using his body. Being a man of great worth, if you are able to manage your sexual desires and control your sexual desires, women won't have any influence over your sexuality. Because sexual desire is a woman's only source of the power.

* Women's Victim Mindset Of Manipulation

Women's victim mentality tends to be disapproving. Women can be very adept at playing the victim. They're never right. They try to view any bad event as not being their fault and passing the blame on to others. If she finds ways to blame someone else to blame her actions and actions, she'll. If she finds an excuse to not feel guilty then she'll. The woman is averse to taking the idea of being held accountable and hates to be responsible. Women don't like taking the responsibility for their actions, and they are reluctant to acknowledge their mistakes and are so resentful of being blamed for something or getting confronted in a negative manner that often they'll attack, whether towards you or anyone else nearby, regardless of whether the information being shared is honest or reasonable. The reputation of women is paramount. It's more important for her than any moral issue, law or principle abstract.

It's all about being in a place where she isn't considered a failure, no matter how damaging and demeaning her way of life is. They do not want anybody who is out there to look behind their cloak of the mystique of their statue. They cover up their tracks, and then manipulate their victims.

Women's truth can be whatever she desires for it to be. If an abstract truth does not meet her needs, a dissociative truth will be created as a substitute.

Do not trust women. Being manipulative and liars can be a threat to their determination and perseverance is for us, our tools in the world.

Men manage interactions by not being reactive; women manage interactions by acting extremely emotional, dramatic, and intense.

* Some Common Victim Mindsets.

-False Tears

It's a very popular woman's victim principle that women use. It's very simple for women to cry (crocodile tears). To make a scene of sympathy her gland of tears to let out tears. When she is able to see tears, a majority of people think she's the one who is suffering.

I was able to build my entire life around him. I was there even when he was poor. I was a victim of his and he would dump me.

In the event that no one was forced into doing anything at their own will by pressure, nobody was harmed.

-Excuses

The woman makes up absurd excuses in order to her feel like a victim, even though she's incorrect.

He didn't pay attention and i was able to cheat, I didn't intend to do it this, but it was just a small error, but I was just foolish.

It is possible to cheat. It was just an opportunity to get away with it. If the guy were to lavish her with attention, she'll still being complaining about the fact that he has become too dependent and apathetic.

Following a few rounds, she'll declare that she was coerced or manipulated. Nowadays, pornstars have started to claim victimhood, saying they were either naive or forced in their entry into the porn scene.

The idea that men can manipulate women into having sex can be an act of manipulation. They wish to appear like they're the victimized so that the public won't consider them to be slutty and unwise. The technique of manipulation is known as "victim entrapment manipulation "

I was sexually molested

It's as shocking as it might seem. Females who do not want to get slutty can become victimization by saying that a man sexually assaulted them. This is especially true if they realize they're not virgins. That's how far women will do to protect her face.

The men see us as sex objects

It's a mentality of victimization. Girls will wear provocative clothes and post pictures of her body via social media sites, and protest at men who aren't liking her.

However, men also are portrayed as objects of ridicule by women. They view males in a negative light. They see men as "success objects". They will label a man aged 20 or older as broke and irresponsible, or without a any future. That's objectification!

The men are players.

They say it all the time in order to make men considered cheaters in general. However, in reality, women are more prone to cheating than women. The reason is that women are less careful and shrewd to get found guilty.

If men cheat, what are they cheating with? stones? Do men cheat with women? This means that women also cheaters.

Chapter 5: The Alpha Male - Masculine Man

Simply put, eing alpha.

is being male means being masculine in all its manifestations. A male who is an alpha man who is a success whatever he chooses to pursue. He recognizes his own worth and conducts things in his personal style, so he pays his attention on himself. He doesn't worry about the opinions of others. He's red pilled and knows the ethos (he isn't displaying his beliefs, but merely follows the rules) Alphas shouldn't boast about that he's red pilled. The actions speak louder than the words. Man is an alpha by the way in which behaves when he takes TRP. It is clear who you are and you don't need to prove your worth or get acceptance. A true alpha isn't looking for recognition, so you don't need to make statements or behave with a specific way to get anyone to love you. It is a fact that how you show the way you want to be what people see of your image and even if they do not agree with you, it's not a big issue. You are liked by people and that's all that matters.

Contrary to popular belief the definition of an Alpha is not someone who works out (muscled) or looks attractive or is a fat person. The term "alpha" refers to the principles, not by physical characteristics.

A true alpha is aware of what he desires from himself and life, and will take whatever steps necessary in order to attain it. He is a person who speaks up is a man who owns his wishes without guilt or shame, establishes clear boundaries, and stands about them when they're violated. Being an Alpha it is your goals, not the needs of an individual woman's, the top first priority. Be a rebel and don't follow her rules adhere to your own guidelines. Enhance your strengths while minimizing your weaknesses. You must not appear vulnerable and regardless of the situation, never be afraid to let her go'.

Do not show weakness as women enjoy pinning on weaknesses of males. Do you think that sharing your weaknesses shows love and trust and that it is possible to connect over your struggles? are wrong. What she is seeing is your vulnerability as repulsive. She doesn't care about the weakness of your soul, or your suffering and how hard to express your feelings to her. Women do not care. They may admire your tenacity against such and adversity, but they don't have to show it.

Do not talk about a woman and you'll end up giving the woman psychological tools to employ against you when you're a victim of shits.

Your weakness will be used against you in order to gain the advantage. When a woman feels that the man she loves is superior to her, then he's visible sexually, but only after the woman believes that a man is superior to her does he appear.

They want men who demonstrate power in a manner which makes them feel superior. If women feel superior to men, she will be drawn to the man. It is important to display your power and control over any circumstance. Women can be controlling and always be in a position to dominate. They'll fight to keep control over the relationship however, once they have it they're unhappy and switch to a different man.

This is a continuous test that and you can't be a failure if you wish to continue your relationship with the woman you're in dispute. When her power increases within the relationship, her admiration and appreciation to you will decrease. When a woman is in a relationship with one of the less powerful men who is trying to dominate and dominate, she'll utterly reject the man. He has accepted that she is submissive so enjoys the power that her control grants her. If he gains power and she becomes a victim, she will lose the power and the resources that her monopoly has allowed her. In addition, she'll never be able to forget the old ways of doing things, she won't ever truly think he's a good chief.

Being an Alpha it is important to not be unpredictably, otherwise people (especially women) could be able to observe your actions and make plans for the future. Don't be open about your motivations. You're better off being perceived as intriguing and entertaining instead of boring and predictable. That's the key to entertaining and humorous conversations with women. You need to keep her guessing at the next step in all of her life as you manage to keep up with sensible and effective activities. Females are drawn to the simplest of things, since it corresponds to their feelings. In order to keep her interested do not divulge all of your secrets to her. If she gets easily familiar with the game, the card will make her bored and she'll seek out fun at a different location.

Cut your cards into pieces. Feed her every piece. The more she is attempting to fix the pieces into an uninteresting picture and the more she is fascinated by the puzzle that lies before her. Women already possess a an affinity for mystery and the dark and mysterious, she won't stop until she has figured out the mystery. The game is played by an alpha.

If you're understood, then you're not attractive. If you are trying to help women get to know you better, and they'll lose trust in your work, and you're making things easier for them to lose respect. Women only value the things they put into their lives, be it the attention of others, commitment or even resources.

Being alpha means discarding your beta traits. Alphas should never act as the beta. In the same way, a beta may not be considered an alpha, nor show alpha movements.

An alcoholic will make the happiness of women his top main goal, even when the simp isn't happy. He will commit actions to his own expense to impress women.

On contrary, doesn't seem to want to be happy. Alphas seek their satisfaction first. He is focused on himself even when it is perceived as selfish.

The simp is in love every day. His wife is the center of his deplorable life. He devotes his valuable (but very limited) time and energy to women, even when they do not respect his. Alpha limits his acceptance. The alpha focuses his energy and energy on building his own. Women receive little recognition even after displaying good behavior and meeting his requirements and desires.

Simps view women as queens, and therefore they are submissive to the women. He strives to help and treat them as special but gets treated like slaves. Alphas view the humans as human beings, thus treating the people as they would treat other humans and does not elevate their status.

Women don't care if you're a good person. They want to know that you've got dominating alpha characteristics to make them feel a little. The alpha will always strive to improve himself. The alpha pays attention to himself since he knows that his worth.

Concentrate on your own. If you develop yourself the same way as men do who respect honour, respect power, vitality and integrity, as well as power as well as status, wealth as well as confidence, body knowledge, wisdom, and experience and experience, you'll be in a position to exercise the strategic control and lead. It's the reason you are the alpha.

Know that life is like a game. You are either playing or you're playing. You must control it. Be a player and don't let the game dictate your actions. Don't be a jerk and don't do things in opposition to your own will. Be honest with yourself and don't be in a hurry to please your friends and family. The concept of humility is deceitful. Be honest with yourself, but do not make decisions that could hurt other people.

Take care of your money, time and your attention. Your health and well-being must be the top priority.

Do not give into pressure. Learn to deal with pressure. Keep your cool and don't be in a rush. Take control of your feelings. This takes some time, however for a man, being emotionally charged is where you are easily manipulated.

Don't be Idle. Your time is valuable and use it to the best of your advantage it is available. Utilize your time to develop yourself up to an level. Don't make use of your time for chasing women. At the end you'll be without a ring to commit yourself to. Avoid chasing women! The way you interact with them is likely to make them want more if you are playing your cards correctly.

Disregarding a woman after having shown her how much fun makes your attractive. If she isn't chasing you away, then leave. If nobody chases you, improve your interpersonal interactions. Be fun to spend time with. Be ready to give up.

* How To Know You Are An Alpha

- You are able to keep eye contact the duration of conversations with others. You're confident and you are not timid. Your speech is more confident.

You decide what rules you want to follow. What people's opinion matters to you than a tiniest bit.

- You view you as the prize, and females as passive players playing the game of dating to be wooed or enticed. Not identical equalists who have to be negotiated into a contract.

It is not a sign of any weakness or show signs of the pain. Accept pain and make it an energy source that keeps striving to reach your objectives. The people who are able to harness their pain have more power than those who seek to hide it out of anxiety.

You don't have a problem walking on your own. Do not be afraid to go on a walk by yourself, rather avoid walking mindlessly in the crowd. You should be a lonely wolf (alpha) but not an insular sheep (beta).

You don't pursue women if they're giving you more than you're worth. You take them off.

You make your time into as a resource and put it to use.

You set boundaries and steer clear of unnecessary debates and individuals who could provoke or test you. You are aware of when you should ignore. Learn when to smile to avoid trouble, and the right time to remain silent to stay clear of trouble. Be strategically. When it comes to life, you must know the right time to quit persevere, the things that merit your time and time, so that you stay out of"sunk costs" "sunk cost effect".

You are able to avoid being controlled and even played.

- You are less open of bullshit generally. You believe in your self-esteem and place yourself at the top. This is what makes you masculine.

Chapter 6: The Female Ideology Of An Alpha - A Real Man

Ask a woman for a description the characteristics of an alpha male the definition of an alpha male, sit in a chair and listen to her talk about the kind of man who will worship and prioritize her needs. It's likely that she'll declare, "an alpha is a faithful man, an alpha should focus attention and be available for his woman, an alpha should spend on me and meet my needs, an alpha should forget a woman's past" or something similar.

In the description of her Alpha, all the attention is focused on her and what the man could do to her. When women refer to "real man", you'll find that they have no idea about what a man actually is. Just a misguided idea of what you can do to help her and accept more of her absurdities.

Have you ever heard women say:

An honest man will place himself first?

Men are expected to go to the gym and appear healthy and attractive to himself?

The real man must invest his time in building his own self?

The real thing is that a man is expected to conduct DNA tests on his children?

The real man must not be spending a lot of money on women?

The real men are expected to investigate an individual's history and examine her with rigor prior to a long-term engagement?

You now have an idea of who the real men really are, and also the message I just delivered.

The real men, the gentleman ideal man, etc. are all terms used by females and sexually oriented society to remind that man to shame him to fulfill women's needs. Remember this!

Do not trust women who is trying to instruct males how to behave. They will only influence you in ways that will benefit you to the detriment of. She believes that a genuine man is that of a simp who's in her hands and at her disposal. She is looking for her own version of an alpha whom she would like to transform into treating as the queen. A person she can use to fulfill her desires. She is looking for a man who has some power and yet she perceives his status as an Alpha i.e she claims you're an actual man, but in actual fact, you're only being deceived.

Females want Alphas who be awed by them. This is why they prefer betas but want fun and thrills with Alphas. They seek qualities that don't reflect the status as an Alpha. They would like a man to never stop spending time with their phones, contact them each hour of the day, make their payments, unlock the doors to them, praise them and pay them respect.

The men that women label unwholesome, patriarchal, and misogynistic are precisely the kind that they marry and date (if they want to) as well as keeping the average male (simp real man) as their male bestie and friendship zone.

If you act as if she's wearing a crown she'll treat you as clowns. If you give her too much attention and you'll be a target for rejection. When you behave as the queen you'll be not seen. Make her feel like a famous She'll treat her like an admirer.

When a woman refers to an individual "narcissistic bully, misogynist, an asshole, a jerk" It's because he's not executing in accordance with her standards. It's just a matter of being an alpha. He's not even the real male.

Congratulations! Congratulations! You're doing everything right. You're inexorable. The manipulation she has isn't working with you the way she'd like. This makes her angry since she is resentful of seeing her doing it. You'll be able to play an innocent victim to you, saying "you don't know how to treat a lady right".

Do not give into her or else she'll manipulate you and manipulate you into becoming an alpha female. Do not bend your rules in order to please her.

It's impossible for her to interact by bringing a male version of herself. Perhaps only for the purpose to get attention, resources as well as emotional support and affirmation easily.

If a woman keeps telling you that "You don't act like a Man" Well, congratulations man You're a winner! You keep thwarting her manipulative scheme. It's an attempt to intimidate men into submitting to her demands. DON'T GIVE IN.

Do you wonder why if women ask you for money, and you are unable to pay her, she labeled the person "a stingy man that doesn't act like a real man" Is she trying to cause you to feel shame (a kind of psychological blackmail that is a result of her desire to control your) to make you feel the at ease being described as "stingy and not a real man" and will give you cash.

If a woman says to that you should "man up" , "be a man for once", "you are not a real man", "you are behaving like a child" or " you are not a gentleman" Just be aware the possibility of manipulation about to happen. The woman is trying to trick to make you believe that you're being less manly which is why she wants the effort to meet her expectations by complying with her requirements and becoming the real supoosed man she's looking for.

Do not try to slim down yourself to the woman's preferences and needs. A man who is an alpha has his own standards, while a man follows his guidelines.

Do not let the idea of being an alpha destroy you and if you are the type of woman she is in the present, then tomorrow she'll seek another flavor and the cycle continues. For a man change for the benefit of women but not for improvement and growth which is beneficial for you can be extremely disruptive. It's no superior than a pawn on the board of chess.

Men aren't liked by women because they can easily be manipulated, moulded and manipulated because they signify weak self-esteem or confidence, and lack of ambition. Instead, she would prefer an individual who is able to quickly enter his frame to create a specific structure.

Make sure you have a sturdy and well-known frame. You shouldn't allow her to mold your. Instead, mold her into the leader of excellence you are and she'll never stop wanting to be.

BRIFFAULTS LAW AND HYPERGAMY

* BRIFFFAULTS LAW

The female is not the

Male determines the aspects that affect the animals in their family. If the female is unable to gain none benefit from the association with males, then there is no chance for such an association to take place.

It means that the past benefits that men receive do offer any guarantee of a the possibility of a future relationship. The men are disposable when woman decides to quit the man she has been with, she'll ignore all advantages she received. According to Briffault's law, females are only able to associate with males and can always benefit from.

For instance, when a man gifts the woman an iPhone as well as expensive clothes but it does not cement her position in the relationship and she is able to choose to walk away if he cannot offer the most current iPhone or fashionable clothes to her.

The woman doesn't have any concern about what a guy has done to her yesterday. She is only concerned about what a man could provide for her in the future and today.

Also, any sacrifices made in the past are unenforceable if the ongoing relationship does not offer her any tangible advantage.

For simplicity: If you can't help her right now it doesn't matter about whether you assisted her prior to. It is not possible to put a woman on a monthly wage and then decide to end it later, and then expect she will not be excited over being with your. The woman will leave once you've stopped giving. The woman will search to find a man who will meet the needs of her present.

The agreement in which males provide a present advantage in exchange in exchange for the promise of the future, is null unenforceable once the male has given the benefits.

The promise of a future benefit is not able to influence future relationships, but the effect is being proportional to the amount of time that will pass before the reward will be granted and related to the degree that the female is trusting male.

What does this mean is that the man who promises the woman about a future reward, can only influence the woman based on trust and duration until she realizes that benefit. The question is, in essence, how long is she required to wait until he makes the payment or pays out, and what is the likelihood that to be able to make the payment. It is an example of deferred gratification as well as probability which can be compared to a choice, in which women must perform for the sake of ensuring that her husband will be able to pay out.

This is usually shown by simps and orbs as they offer positive benefits for females, however they do not receive advantages of an upcoming relationship. Males are viewed by their reproduction capacity in the same way as Beta Bucks with no benefit accrued from themselves.

Then they discover they've been discarded and used in the trash - the discarded sexual sex. It is a way to meet her needs for self-gratification.

* HYPERGAMY

"Higher-gamy" or hypergamy" is the term applied to the practice or habit of who is married to a partner of a more social or caste status that they.

For females the female desire to get married to the most beautiful woman she can get. This is due to an intrinsic genetic desire to be a mother with the highest quality of genes. Females are drawn to men who are bigger than they and smarter than their peers make more money over them, is more fun than them, and more powerful than them, etc. It is the nature of women to be attracted by men who are equal or above her. Hypergamy in women is bipolar, meaning that you're either superior or inferior. If a woman views she is superior to a male she is invisible sexually and only when she considers that a man is superior his image become apparent.

If she's in a relationship with an individual, if she meets a man who is better than her man, and she is attracted to her, she'll leave her boyfriend for someone else This is Branch in motion.

The women are drawn to people who have more value over them. That's the reason they're very highly sexually oriented. So long as they're able to be sure to branch their swings towards an individual with more value the majority of them are likely to do it. They'll justify it with the notion that love has gone between the two of you. They'll say "we just lost vibes, the love is no longer as strong as it used to be". That's a shame! It's not true! This is a method to get rid of yourself in order to gain the man with more value. It is a common practice to seek out those who can surpass their own.

They want men who demonstrate power in a way which makes them feel less powerful. If a woman is feeling less than a male then she becomes attracted to his appearance - this is the reason women are extremely attracted to signs of standing (good genes as well as wealth, confidence the status of others). It can be manifested in a variety of ways. The most well-known is the gold-digging; and being attracted to a person exclusively because of his financial wealth.

For understanding the concept of hypergamy it is necessary to have a good understanding of SMV. SMV is a term used to describe the value of sexuality. All people, female and male has SMV.

How Is SMV Measured?

It is determined through the analysis of anything that has anyone worth. The things that make humans valuable are the following: beauty, wealth and skills, as well as talent fame, glory, and humor. It is all that's beneficial for any human which other human beings can admire.

For men and a sexually attractive one, the more your market value is, the more attractive you are and the harder it gets to get rid of your. Nevertheless, you're still disposable.

If we were to determine the SMV for women. If from a total of 10, we award the woman 5 points to be beautiful, 5 to the riches of her life, five for skill and the list goes on. Her SMV is the sum from all of them, which is 5. Therefore, her sexual market value will be 5 out of 10. She will choose men who have an SMV 5 or higher however not less than 5.

There is another person we can have. It's a male this time. When he is rated the value of his score is calculated at 8. Thats 8/10

The concept of hypergamy is straightforward. We'll look at it from a different angle. The man scored 8, while the female scored 5.

The SMV of his is extremely excessive, but take a take a look at his SMV of 5. The woman's SMV isn't even close. It is possible that she scores high on elegance, but is a bit low on other measures but the guy can be so low in his commitment to the girl, and perhaps feel proud of her!

This is men who are for you.

Let's flip the situation. In the event that the female scored the same than the man, while the male scored at least as lower as her and the woman was never to be able to date him. It's called female hypergamy.

The woman she loves will never accept lower. Her search is always for men who have greater SMV that she. She is never in a lower level.

The fact that females are constantly looking for men with more value, whereas men don't really care is something we refer to as female hypergamy.

An affluent man may see the beauty of a woman with small SMV and choose to get married her. Apart from beauty, she's worthless in any way. If you take SMV into account her scores are extremely low when compared to male. If people discuss the wedding, they do not consider it is because he created a woman who was likely to live in poverty to become wealthy. The beauty of her is not important as you consider the value of what he has contributed to the marriage!

In the context of this we can conclude that a largely untried factor in the female sexual inclination to hypergamy is only possible due to men are naturally able to help it grow. In any society, for instance the men naturally organize themselves into a an order of competency, and females will pick men who are dominant in the highest position of that the order. The woman has nothing to have to do with hierarchical structures and she is just looking for the most delicious cut of meat from it.

Women are known to be extremely sexually active, and that is the reason they strive to find the best companions they have the ability to. One of the easiest ways to determine "higher quality" is by comparing mates.

First guy drives a benz while the other driver drives the Bugatti. The second guy is the winner.

The first guy is strong and the and the second one has abs. The second man wins.

First guy is funny and has a sense of humor. Second man is well-known. The second guy is the winner. Etc

Women prefer men who are superior to other men. This shouldn't be an issue for the person you are. In the course of time, she'll start dating new men, and not just to one prior partner, but rather with all her friends. He was a successful man, a well-known or a great guy and if you do not perform well in any of the three of these categories, she believes she's not worthy of higher. The subconscious comparison is starting to compare yourself to other guys and she'll be upset if you do not rock her as each of them did. A strong male defended her, while the popular guy makes her popular, etc.

Bitter truth right? The knowledge i have shared would not be harsh or bitter, I just said that it would be the reality.

Women are innately incapable to love the way men do. And they are not able to love, i.e unconditional love is a joke. Women appreciate opportunism and constantly seek out the best choice.

Behind every successful person is an attractive woman.

Women aren't interested in the struggles you face, they only care about your accomplishments. They are looking for the end result. However, successful men appreciate women who have been there through the entire process. Women hate risk, which is why they are prone to stifle ambitious men by expressing their fearful insecurity.

The women are drawn to the wealthy. A man's wealth appears similar to makeup on women. The makeup of money is for males. It's what draws women.

As i mentioned earlier I am not a fan of it the moment men set themselves up in high value and find themselves with a female with a very lower SMV. Do not settle to less. In general, women don't want to settle for lesser. Males should be following the same fashion. The days where men who have large SMV are able to grab women who has lower SMV and offer her the world. Ladies wouldn't be doing you a favor, no matter how many billions they own. It's not a matter of hatred It's just a matter of the right manner of treatment. This is the age of gender equality and feminism, which women long for so long.

Chapter 7: What Can A Lady Offer You

You may think that she's worth it

since all she can provide is appearance and a genital?

I'd like you to be more aware!

The red pill makes women realize that they don't have anything to offer other beyond their bodies. They are aware of this because they're constantly looking good and highlighting the one real assets they can use to get by.

However, in the words that come out of the mouth, only a handful of women are willing to admit that they're just an excuse to cover up an array of fuckholes due to the fact that the process of "dehumanisation" harms their ego and erodes the essence of what they really are. Narcissism is the very thing they seek to reinforcing and reinforce through external validation from social media (cue dopamine screams in the form of Instagram filtering selfies and facebook likes, and the refusal to take down a phone) and a meticulous regimen of applying makeup and carefully selected clothes.

Women are not happy when confronted with "what they have to offer" But should you request them to provide you with something of value, all they're suffering from is their bodies.

Who do they see twerking in music videos? Who is showing their boobs and butts on the internet? It's likely to be women.

It is true that women are known to dress in provocative ways, show their nakedness on the internet, and later, they protest that they're considered sexy objects.

The way they behave is like a sexual object, however they become annoyed when they're treated as a sex subject. Women recognize that their greatest assets are their sexuality and beauty. But then they are able to crucify males for believing they are the same.

The Patrice O'Neal Test

"Ladies, how would you keep your man if you lost your vagina?" The late comic Patrice O'Neal often asked the audience. If women were always responding by expressing sexual arousal and oral sexual activity, O'Neal would say, "See, I gave the opportunity to speak about yourself and now you're an assortment of holes. You're supposed to be treated like a special person, but you're really simply an assortment of holes to your self."

The same thing happened when O'Neal asked the question to the audience. The comedian was hilarious, but an awake man is aware of that he's right.

Women are aware of how correct she is despite their attempts to disbelieve that.

If they are given the opportunity of bringing something new in the room, aside from the sex industry, women instantly transform their bodies into sexual objects.

If you ask a woman what she can offer you in the way of marriage apart sexual intimacy. Once she's completed talking about the heavens and earth (you are aware of what I mean) then, you should inform her that you're not getting married. What's more, the very next question she'll pose will be one (or in connection with) this;

How do you fulfill your sexual desire? The answer is simple: sexual sex.

-How do you get children? The answer is still tied to sexual sex.

It is obvious that she will never be willing to accept women's is only interested in sex. Yet she's still asking what you'll do to get sex while trying to be a parent when you tell she you're not getting married.

In the event that you and two other ladies at in this moment are engaged in an exchange in which one of them declares that she's not planning to get married and the very first question that the other lady might ask her would be among (or a part of) the following:

Who will take care of your kids? (Notice: She did not inquire about who be the birth mother however, she asked who to look after your children, meaning that they are aware that children can originate from any place they like but the money needed to support them must come from a steady source)

Who would care for your needs when you're old (still is a matter of cost).

They would not be asked questions such as: what would you contribute the value of? whom could you be able to help develop and who you would be blessed by? And other qualities women say they provide in the marriage.

Chapter 8: Female Nature, Hyper Gamy And Female Genitals

What is it that women really want? This is a question all men would like to know. Women are wired with a feminine nature. It is referred to as Hypergamy. It is the feminine instinct to search for a husband who can be at or more in sexual attraction and financial assets. If you search all around, it is extremely difficult to locate women who are dating at a lower level than their market worth. Take, for instance, a take a look at the nurse. What is the most frequent instance of nurses who are female dating doctor? Most of the time and yet how often you find an female doctor with a male nurse? Most likely, never. Similar to female paralegals. They are more likely to meet a lawyer than a male paralegal within the same field. Women who date men who are at the same level or more is due to the desire to keep their standard of living when they are ready to have children as they're likely to be less productive when they have a child. Women who work in jobs that require white collars are less likely to date males working in blue collar positions. There is a lot of women who want to meet an enviable number of males. The next step is to discuss both genders and how they complement one with respect to the traditional relationship.

Masculine & Feminine - Preselection

Both genders seek different things when it comes to relationship and dating. Females look for traits that are masculine while men look at feminine traits. The men look for women that are a great mom and wife. Females look for Men with confidence, and have the ability. They rank these traits very high since competent men are able to care to their families in the event of having children. Every woman who gets older are likely to seek out men with the financial stability. If you are financially prosperous, you'll enjoy more opportunities with females and get picked for preselected. This type of selection is what folks consider to be a very valuable man. There are very few males today who belong in this category however once you're in the group, in the group, you'll have the freedom to select and pick who you like. Then let's look at the two kinds of guys that women love to date.

Beta and Alpha Men - Attraction Levels

There are two varieties of men. They are known in the terms Alpha as well as Beta. These are opposite ends from the same spectrum. Beta is the male whom women consider to be being the primary caregiver, whereas Alpha is viewed as a male who is considered to be the best potential father. The two differ on a number of levels and most men aren't on either of these sides. The majority of males are at the middle. Personally, I think it's more beneficial to consider it as three different levels. The three tiers are average, over-average and below the average. Make an honest look at your position on the attractiveness scale. It is good to know that the majority of men are able to change this and improve their worth by either improving their financial situation or by changing their appearance. Women also tend to search for different things as they age. They are likely to look for various characteristics as they grow older and search for the long-term relationship. If you are a man that has become extremely valuable in the short-term or long-term partner of women, it is your choice whether you want to be in an intimate relationship or remain single. Do not let someone force you to take a decision in the direction of their desires rather than your own. Make sure you are the first to make a choice and resist the advice of others that tell you that you must marry without being prepared. You are the one to decide whom you would like to marry rather than your family or friends. your family.

Masculinity and Leadership Roles In Relationships

What do women want? Every guy is looking for answers to. It's simple. The women want a man who is a leader as well as the one who provides for the relationship. In a relationship that is traditional women are looking for men who have the ability to take decisions. They do not just need to take choices here and there and to be able to believe that they are capable in the long term. Women do not like males who constantly ask for their opinion when making choices. There is always one who is dominant and the other submissive within a relationship. The majority of men aren't happy being the person who decides and have been taught that women have to be the ones who approve of all things. Let me provide an illustration. Imagine that you're going to take one of your friends on a date for the first time. There's no way to know what food she enjoys or if she might be sensitive to certain food items and therefore you need to inquire about what she'd prefer to consume. Another option and a simple way for this is to offer her two options. This way, she won't be stressed before going out on the date. Another method is to take her out to a bar and keep things easy. This can be acceptable for the first date. However, If you asked questions on the next date then she'd begin to be angry as she thinks you're not in a position to take the final choice without her consent. It's going be a bit absurd, but ladies want that you "get it". They want you to take the lead. They do not want to show you how to leadership role, they want you to follow their lead since they think that it's a natural characteristic for men to make plans for their dates. They don't just want you to be able to organize your dates, but they also do nothing to instruct you on. They are skills learned during dating, but eventually if not yet there, you'll learn from the experience of others, so don't fret even if you don't possess those abilities as of now.

How Modern Dating Works-Meeting Women-Attraction-Are You Her First Choice

The modern dating scene is more different from traditional dating 20 to 30 years ago. Today, in the world of dating, it is essential to keep up with modern times. It is essential to meet new people on the internet, in person and even via your friends or your circle of friends. However, it's not as simple as it seems. The majority of women reject guys they meet on dating websites. On tinder it's even worse. Females reject 95 percent of people they meet through Tinder. Tinder dating application. How do you overcome this and be one of Tinder's most desirable males? First, hiring the services of a professional photographer. When you find a lady who has posted pictures online, it's likely that she's shot anywhere from 50 to 100 photos in order in order to create the ideal image she's going to upload. In order to make yourself make yourself stand out it is essential to hire an experienced photographer. This is something that many men aren't doing. It is important for your photos to make an impression, which is why you are the most sought-after man when it comes to online dating. Additionally, you would like to be with women you're drawn to. It is not worth engaging in relationships with women you don't have a desire for and those who show little interest in you. In the future, we'll examine desires and the way they affect relationships, but at this point we'll concentrate on the fundamentals. Think about it when you're in the middle of a date. Do you think she is my top choice? If there was a big crowd of women standing before you, and she was in the group Would you pick her over others? It's a question to think about. Take a look at the way she's acting during the day. Do you think she is in a hurry to get home, or do she wish to prolong the date? We will then be discussing more specific factors to be looking for in dates that show that she is interested in your. Be aware that you are under no obligation to attend. The purpose of the event is to meet one person and find out whether there's any connection. If the person you're meeting with displays an absence of respect or disrespect for either you or the time that you spend with her it is best to terminate the date before. Don't tolerate bad behaviour from females, particularly during the first meeting.

Chapter 9: Attraction Level And Hyper Gamy

Are they not in your zone? What is your position in the scale of attraction? It is important to be aware of before beginning to date. There must be a fair assessment of your position on the market for dating. Everyone evaluates you on 1-10 on a scale. It is important to know the difference between women who see your character as average, above average or less than average. This is an excellent indicator of the kind of woman you'll attract. If you're not certain what you are doing There are apps for free that allow users to assess your images so you'll have an concept of if you're representing your self well. The nature of women is to search for a man who has the same or more with respect to earnings as well as physical attractiveness, work or educational levels. In other words, if she earns 50k a year, she'll be seeking men who make an average of at least 50 thousand per year or more since in the end, she would like your ability to meet her needs in the event you have to work more or less. If there's an difference in income, it could result in problems for relationships, particularly in the event of a sudden shift in lifestyle or finances because of the economic situation. People in relationships that last for a long time are looking for financial security. So, when you begin to fall behind in your financial situation and begin earning less than she does then she may think about whether you're competent enough to be able to start an entire family. There is nothing to get upset over. This is how women function. Additionally, there's an important distinction between someone who simply wants to get your sources, but is not able to establish the emotional connection, or is a materialist. These women aren't ideal for long-term relationships and you must avoid these types of women. If you're with an ongoing relationship with a partner who you get fired and she is unable to accept that you'll come back. Be the leader, since if she has to step from her comfortable space to be the leader and become the feminine woman, she'll begin to be resentful of you due to your mistakes. Learn to recognize which side of the psychological attraction scale, and understanding how hypergamy impacts the relationship you have with your partner. It is inevitable that you will experience some ups and downs but you'll never be defeated by all issues.

Why Men who are less attractive become Wanty: Women always compare them to other relationships.

There are certain types of men who are only interested in romance? Yes. They are the men who aren't aware of their options or aren't aware of have a lot of options in the market because they're afraid to move or risk the possibility of meeting people new because of the risk of being turned down. In the past there are women who only view males as a source of support which is why you must be wary of such women. In particular, she has children. The need for a caretaker will be because that her ex-partner is not getting along with her. The relationships that are formed can result in catastrophe because women who are like this can be prone to ignoring any sort of signals that indicate attraction and make unrealistic demands of your role as a caretaker even though it shouldn't be your obligation. One way to establish the stage for a romantic relationship is by attracting and, if you're a man is to ensure her to meet your requirements. A different thing women tend to do is look at relationships in comparison. The way they compare their relationships with the ones who surround her, including relatives and friends. Then, she will seek their endorsement to determine the if you're an appropriate option to her. For a man, you must avoid any suggestions from the people she has referred to as her acquaintances. You and your spouse to decide what you'd like to achieve in your relationship. Take note that your partner may offer advice that could result in your being a slave within the relationship. It is also possible that they will give you negative advice due to the fact that they don't wish to see you as a couple, so be sure to take everything that everyone else around you is saying with a pinch of salt. The relationship is an important status symbol for females. There is always a competition against each other to determine who's doing best. Ladies always want to feel confident that they've found the right man especially in her close friends.

Women's Decline in Looks - Dating Market Value

The value of a woman's relationship is dependent on the value of her sexuality. The market value of a woman isn't solely based on appearance however, it also depends on how she enhances your life. Females peak at 20-years-olds with regard to attractiveness, several studies have revealed. As men age and become more attractive, women rate a 20-year old as the being the most appealing. The values begin to decline when they reach their 20s. That's why lots of women want for marriage at a young age regardless of what the media claims. The majority of women know they're in the midst of a fetus timer and after thirty, it goes downwards each year. The ideal time to meet women for relationships is between the ages of 24-26. Females will choose to date men who are slightly older than them, with expectation that he's more mature and skilled than those of her in their twenties. The value of a man's relationship increases as he grows older. People in their 30's have greater options for dating than their earlier years due to the fact that they must create value when they grow older. They need to be able to take care of their children and family. The women who date older men are expected to do this. They are not looking for a shabby guy who is in his 30's. Especially when they are higher educated and make higher than the average male. It is important to build up your worth. It is possible to date younger women than you, if you've built worth to yourself. Women are able to choose their partners at the age of late 20's, but they only have a short duration of time because of the window of fertility for being able to have children. The best man can be the men in the top 10% and pick the person you like instead of someone who you are required to choose since you didn't have a choice.

Chapter 10: The Party Girl - Setting Boundaries

Is it normal for a girl to drink out when she's engaged or has children? There is no need to say. The sole reason why she'll be out in public is if she's in the mood to party or wants to get praise from men. In either case, it's not a good idea for relationships. It's not uncommon for many women to enjoy a girls' nights out, however it's also quite common for a large percentage of these women to divorced or to get divorced in the near future. Keep an eye out for buddies who would like to regularly invite her to bars or a nightclub. It is something that needs to be addressed during the initial stages of an affair. Drinking in bars is something you shouldn't accept. You should inform her quickly to her peers and make sure they be respectful of her rules. If this continues to happen or if she decides for a night out with group of friends despite your wishes You must recognize that you're being snubbed. Someone who feels the desire to party even when in a relationship probably an impulse-driven person. Perhaps you're wondering "how to do I set these boundaries?" It is important that they are set prior to becoming intimate. A lot of people make the error of trying to discuss the boundaries once they're involved in a relationship. However, they usually don't work smoothly. If she wants to ask to be monogamous, ask her what she's looking to find in a partner. Then she will inquire about the same thing and then you will make your requirements public. What topics to discuss is the most crucial issues. There will be a time when she tests the boundaries. Make it clear the things you would like to see in the relationship, and she must adhere to your instructions. If she violates the lines of what you expect, it could be time to end the relationship. If the rules of your relationship are well-known and she is still ignoring your rules, then it is best to find an alternative partner who will respect the qualities you can bring to the table.

Women Move on Very Fast - The Family Dynamic

This is a secret to breaking ups and women. Women will move on more quickly than you. This is due to the fact that it's likely that she's had a lot of thoughts about even before breaking off with you. This isn't the only reason for her to break up with you. Perhaps it was because in time, you changed. You was too open and let all the things she needed and turned into a "yes man. Females don't appreciate those who seem too likable. Do not be scared to tell her to stay away. You might get her angry initially however she'll change her behavior in the future. If you force her to punish bad behavior by agreeing to her demands, she'll keep doing it until you've decided enough and said"no. Don't be too surprised when you see a woman break apart with you. A majority of breakups originate from women, just as divorces. In some cases, the issue isn't your fault. The person you are with could be who is uneasy with others. If you're trying to determine the quality of someone with you, check out the parents of her. It's always a great indication. If the parents of her child are in a positive relationship, and her father is the head of the household, the chances are that her partner could replicate the same behaviour. People tend to follow their parents' footsteps. A different tip is to ensure that you have a great connection with her dad. This can be a positive indicator that you respect men. Nowadays, a large number of women aren't from a good families. Pay close to your divorce rates as it is the same over several years. That's due to divorced parents who are more likely to end up divorced when they are adults.

The Steps from Dating to the Relationship

Are you aware of what you are looking for in a woman? Today, most men are ridiculed for their expectations, but don't give in to people who make fun of your character. There are likely to be personal problems and do not want to exclude them from the dating scene. Below are a few criteria you should consider when they are in a relationship. One of them is that she needs to have gotten over her drinking period. It's not like she's in college. This doesn't mean that you can't have dinner with her friends, however, the days of hopping out to bars in a variety of locations ought to be long gone. The second thing is that she must earn money and be employed. Being an adult, she ought to be paying the bills on her own and especially at the first few months of a relationship. Be wary of females that want to get in quick, because it may be done in order to convince you to cover her expenses. Keep in mind that this is a relationship phase. If you're a parent, there are many changes in the family dynamics and she may need be able to work part-time while trying to be a parent however, that's quite a ways off. Thirdly, she is solely focused on her work. It's fine for women who have goals however, someone who prioritizes their work over the relationship or family are probably in a masculine frame and is not the ideal companion. Number four, look at her friends. They're a reflection of her, regardless of whether you're willing be open about it. Are they rude and loud? Take time with your friend to determine if the behavior patterns emerge. I wouldn't be shocked to see these behaviors after 6 months of relationship. Fiveth, does she have a great relation with her dad. Women cannot be in a relationship with a male in the absence of a great relationship with her father as well as an individual she admires. The relationship she shares with her father could be an indication of how she sees and values males. Beware of any woman who have a bad relationship with their father or suffer from constant conflict in their relationships with their families. These are the things you ought to be looking out for. So, will discuss the time what you need to be looking for those. And who is asking for the relationship? As a guy, don't ever solicit a relationship. The result will be the woman making your rules while some women regard the whole thing as completely turning off. One of the people who asks for a relationship holds little influence in the dynamic of the relationship. One of the worst things you can do as a guy is to appear insecure to your woman whom you wish to have to have a romantic relationship with. In the second place, it is important to not be settling down prior to reaching the age of 30. The majority of men reach their professional heights and are more appealing in the 30's and 40's. You don't need to wait for that long however, you must begin dating in the late to mid-30s. At this point, you'll be the most potential value in the world of dating and you can meet someone who is younger than you.

How women can communicate with each other indirectly

Females speak only one language. this is known as indirect communicating. Did you have a relationship with somebody and asked the day's events and she gives brief answer, and then says it was okay? And even more frustratingly, if you observe that she's unhappy regarding something and want to know what's wrong with her, she says that nothing is wrong. If someone you're with says there's nothing not right, there's something not right. Another reason women are demanding men to understand them psychologically. The majority of men aren't aware of the psychology of women and this isn't easy. Have you done something that made her angry at you? It is her expectation that you figure it out. The reason she would like you to understand the issue is to show two points, you are a level of social intelligence when it comes to her needs for emotional support and as well, that you are aware of the primary method women use for communication, which is known as indirect communication. People who know the psychology of females can recognize when it is appropriate to converse and when to leave her time. Indirect communication is the result of her manner of speaking through her body language and how she expresses herself. It is a different way of communicating how men talk because they are able to communicate in a direct manner. If you are looking for something, can ask them to get it. On the other hand, women would like to be able to tell you the way she expresses her emotions herself. This is a difficult task since if she's angry the other day but doesn't wish to talk about it, that's understandable however, if this is a thing that she is prone to doing regularly, then you may want to start dating an alternative person as it may indicate manipulative behavior. It is important to recognize that if you're having a rough day, simply give her space. It will come to chat with you about it. If the same thing happens over and over again you should leave and start dating another person because she's likely to alter her behaviour. It may be a indication of the emotional manipulation she's used with other former relationships.

Chapter 11: Have No Expectations From Women

Don't have any expectations of ladies. If you meet someone online via a dating site or face-to-face and think you may want to meet their profile, the first thing to be able to tell yourself is that she is a normal individual. There is nothing special about her. She doesn't have any obligations to you and are simply getting to know her better to find out whether she can provide you with the same amount of value as you could offer to her. The most damaging thing you can be doing is to get overly excited and look excessively eager. It will cause her to believe that there are no alternatives to dating and can instantly decrease her desire towards your. Many guys make the error of valuing too much what women can offer prior to meeting their potential partner. So, it is important to be able to meet more than one partner as you'll likely invest more when you do not have numerous options for dating. This will give you more confidence and your partner will also be aware. Women are able to tell when males are looking for alternatives or they're desperate and don't have lots of friends to meet. Women already know by how you dress, but also the way you schedule your dates. If, for instance, you ask her to change the date of a date with you and you accept with no hesitation, you give an impression of having no other commitments and are willing to put your money into her, in the absence of her showing her value to you. That doesn't mean you are her only option among the women she would like to select among. The lesson to take away is to not be that man who keeps making calls when the date has ended. Have a fun date. Be relaxed and be open to someone who is right for you.

Female indirect Conversation openers

Are you aware of male acquaintances who are asked out by women? It's not common, however, it happens. The men who are like this are scouted and rank in the top 10-20 percent of attractive men, in the same way as mentioned previously. Females approach males via two different ways: by direct and indirect methods. It's a shame that many men aren't aware of the women who approach them, because they are doing it in indirect ways in order to avoid all forms of rejection. Women hate being rejected. They would rather avoid taking an opportunity to meet someone who could be attracted to her. The best way women approach is when she is chatting about you at a club in close proximity and then flirts with you heavily until it cannot be interpreted as something other than. The woman wants to be with you, and would like to make it known. Not only to you, but also to women you know. You might get her number with no need to ask or take your phone number to phone you back later. Direct conversation openers for females are easy to spot and shouldn't be overlooked. Let's discuss the indirect openers women make to initiate conversations. If a woman is ever able to initiate an exchange with you, it's due to her desire for to be noticed. It's not easy for women to start conversations since men generally are attracted to women. When a woman begins conversations, she's likely to be incredibly attractive to her. One way for her to indirectly communicate with you is through asking you questions which has a non-binding answer and could lead the conversation in another direction. The woman might ask whether you like your pants, or where you're from, or may give you a compliment. The majority of men shun or shrug off such conversations because they're not paying attention, and since this is not often the case that they do not even notice the incident. Another sign of a good relationship is when she is willing to purchase drinks for you. If she's willing to pay for you to drink, it indicates that she is in great attraction to you and believes in your importance. There is also a chance that she thinks that you've got a more attractive market for dating over her. Don't underestimate the woman who is eager to start an exchange with you. It's probably the woman who is looking to invest in you, and she has the potential for you.

Women's Dating Stages By Age

You've been in a relationship lately and asked her what's the longest she's been without a partner? She replies that it's an extended time between her last relationship. She's just being single and focused only on herself. This isn't what you'd like to be hearing. It's true that she's flirting casually without seeking a partner for the long haul. It is crucial to know at what stage women are looking to get married. Women in their university years may not be in search of a long-term relationship. Women who are considered to be relationship capable will begin seeking a relationship that lasts at the age of 24 to 26 and might get married before 28 years old, which is considered to be the median date for marriage within the U.S. But today, many women are awaiting what I refer to as the settling down period to begin looking for a partner who is long-lasting. It is a disadvantage that there are so many women in the same age group that men should concentrate on those in the mid-20's. The time for settling down is between the ages between 27 and 30. The problem arises as women begin to search for a partner who will last a long time around this age, as they're likely to be more involved and most likely to be more eager to get settled. It is not a good thing since women may try to change their behaviour temporarily in your favor and will later reveal to that they're not who they claim to be. A different group of women is in the 30-35 age bracket. This is a group of women you would prefer to avoid. These are probably extremely masculine and are likely to take the lead in their relationships and might already have children from a previous relationship. Women in the last category are older than 35. They are some of the most unhappy women that you encounter. These unrealistic expectations are absurd. The woman will attempt to convince the baby to share with her as soon as you can. She may even be a little grumpy about the fact that she's in a situation in which she's waited all this time to start an infant, even though this isn't your blame. Many women who are dating at the end of their 30's are working women who do not put aside the need to meet a partner for a long time or even have children. This is why it's important to stay with women between the ages of 24-26 because that is the time to meet females who are feminine and seek longer-term relationship.

How can you approach a female to come out, and then set up a date

A common question is what to do when you want to take a woman to go out. Easy. Hi My name is Nick. It's that simple. Keep your cool. Do not be a jerk and a prick. Simply introduce yourself and inform her that you need to start and then inquire for her phone number. Another option is to offer her the number. If she does call you back, it is obvious that she has attractive since she's the person who initiated the conversation, and, consequently, is after you. The next step is setting dates and verifying the date. This is where things can get difficult. Do not give her the place of the date prior to the date. Discuss when you'd prefer to schedule the date and go out to dinner or for a low-risk date as this ensures she won't be under pressure to stay for too long, if you don't get it right. One of the best ways to ensure your date is to give her what time it is early during the day. Then, approximately 1 hour prior to the date, inform her of where to meet. It will lessen the chances of disapproval because if she wants to make changes, it would already have made it clear prior to doing so. A lot of guys commit the error of releasing the date and date in the early stages and phone her to find out whether they're going. It causes uncertainty in her head which causes her to wonder if she really wants to attend. If you hold off to a later date, she'll be waiting that you call her, and inform her of the place she should meet at. What should you expect from your first meeting is a little chat and a bit of flirting. Don't be too serious, and avoid discussing your ex. You should end the date earlier to ensure that it doesn't exceed an hour. It is important to conclude the evening on a positive note and not at the point where conversations become monotonous. If you're still flowing well when you finish your date, she could invite you to her or your location afterward. After the night, most men should take the money, as it's a first time they've met. Thus, it's best to keep the date informal and enjoyable, thus it doesn't add in the end. Don't go out to dinner until after. Of course, some women accept a payment as an attractive gesture, however should she be insistent, you can let her take care of her portion in the event that she would like to. In case you're dating someone who is willing to cover the whole date, then it is an indication of her attraction. It is for her an expression of gratitude for having a great time. Do not turn her down even if she suggests this, as she'll interpret the offer as a refusal. You can invite her to your home for a glass of drinks and have a good time.

What is the best time to keep your distance and what is the best way to meet casually

What is the best frequency to go out with her? About once per every week would be a great idea. If she decides she would like to spend more time with you, she'll let you know and will reach out to you. The majority of women go on between three to five dates to be intimate. Be aware that you are able to and should be dating other people also. This will provide you with more confidence. Women can feel that. They prefer to date a guy to compete for one who doesn't have girlfriends. his. If a man is in the process of dating others has options. One-time relationships with a single woman are considered to be of unimportant. In the process of dating If you have a relationship lasting longer than three to four months, the issue whether you are in a relationship is likely to occur. It's better if she's one who brings it up since it indicates that she's got an interest in getting married and she views yourself as an attractive man. Whichever you decide to do, it's your decision. If you've been with someone for since a long time, you're bound to also like her, so give her a shot if you think you like her and she matches your criteria. What if you do not have a desire to be in a relationship, but you want to remain casually with her? It's possible to lose her, but make sure you keep her within the circle of friends and remain open for a casual rendezvous. Inform her that you value the company of her, however you are too busy to engage in relationships, however you love her and would like to make close friends. When you invite her into the "friend zone," it preserves the possibility of having an informal date to be open since the person who is first to put people in the zone is the most valuable person within the relationship.

Chapter 12: Low Attraction And The No-Contact Rule

You went out on the date, and everything did well however, there's a problem: she's never making contact. This could be a sign that she's an inability to attract her or there was someone else she was looking at before meeting you. It's not your fault. It's possible to have a wonderful date, but at times the lady may have had a relationship with a man prior to you, and are still not in a relationship. If she's not calling back, or is contacting at a lower level and you're not sure if she's interested, then I'd suggest not rushing and letting her call you. If she does not return your call the next step is to confirm that the attraction was not high and you're the only option. The decision not to contact women afterward is a common rule, known as the"no-contact rule. If the woman truly is drawn to you, and you're her primary preference, she'll eventually make contact. If she takes longer to make contact, her hand, the less interest she shows in your persona. This is not the only option. If you are feeling that she is being hesitant, you should make sure to wait for her to contact first, and then you'll discover how attractive her levels are.

She would like to end her relationship

What do you do if engaged but, suddenly is she deciding to end the relationship? This isn't a good thing. This means that she is looking to review her options. You may want to consider what she could do better than you do in the market for dating. This could happen due to various reasons. It could be that she lost weight and was more attractive and began receiving more attention, or was less interested in your physical appearance and emotional. It can be difficult to maintain relationships, but when she decides to rest, it is very likely that she wants to stay with other guys and likely has someone already in her mind who she'd like to meet. Another reason could be that she was given an raise at work but your earnings are less than she does. It will affect the relationship since women tend to look down on men who earn less than they do. A number of studies have demonstrated that. In the long run cannot be tolerant of men who earn less than she does and cannot take care of the family. The reason for this is that financial stress is why many couples end up breaking up. women are looking for financial security after they've reached a certain age, and do not wish to take on the financial burden of the men. When she demands to end your relationship, it is best to immediately start meeting other individuals. It shows her you have value in the marketplace of dating. The primary reason you should start with a relationship as quickly as you can is the fact that women change more quickly than men after an affair ends. The chances are that you will feel miserable when you see her going on dates. Therefore, you should get out with your buddies and make new friends.

She would like to see you again when she has left her

What happens when after an absence, she decides to reunite? Do not ever let her return. If you're married and children, the situation becomes much more complex, however when you do decide to ask her back, she has to be able to prove herself worthy. The majority of relationships that end up breaking up only to re-join with each other don't last over the long term If you do have children then clearly, I can understand why you'd try to come up with a solution. The woman should not be permitted to go back to the house you live in. You're beginning to get married at the start. You're now being chased by her. It's her responsibility to earn it, and you need to establish your own standards. You're in a leadership post and can decide to let her go or not. You know that, too. She will also have a greater respect for you because she perceives you to be someone with a higher relationship market value. Perhaps you're not ready to be able to get her back, and that's what males should do if there's no children present. This is easy to do, simply let her know that you're not. The women in this situation are generally never asked to leave and might be at first astonished or even turned off, but you must stick to the decision since most women have no intention of changing who they are. Let's suppose you've been married for a while but now are seeking divorced. Let me reveal one thing. You will receive all the help from her close friends and perhaps even some of your family members if they're married couple. The majority of men have friends who go through the divorce. The church too will be against her. The thing I've observed is that women always support other women. They're like one-woman groups that protect one another. They will always stand up for each other against males.

Female unicorns: The ideal woman

What's when you think of a unicorn female? Female unicorns are the perfect woman. It is the woman that you've been looking for. Each and every good thing you could think of is a perfect example of she has. No negative behavior which you observe in contemporary women. The woman wants to be a good mother and take care of the home. She is never angry. She does not talk down to the other person. The unicorn even demands that you lead the family without having to ask concerns. It's one of the unicorns in female form. This is an uncommon woman. The majority of men likely will never meet a woman as unique as her. Female unicorns are an ideal for many men. They do exist however it's extremely uncommon to see one. when you encounter women with the traits mentioned above, it's probably the result of knowing they're what you're looking for. The traits listed belong to women of good families, but who they are naturally feminine. They do not constantly make you uncomfortable since their primary interests lie being a mother and raising children. Most women in the present do not come from a stable family and are primarily driven by their careers. It's therefore crucial to eliminate women who do not meet your expectations for those who are willing to become your spouse and to raise your children. Although the unicorn female is extremely rare, you may nonetheless find someone who is long-term by sticking to your rules.

www.ingramcontent.com/pod-product-compliance
Lightning Source LLC
Chambersburg PA
CBHW070556010526
44118CB00012B/1347